Chair Yoga
For
Men Over 50

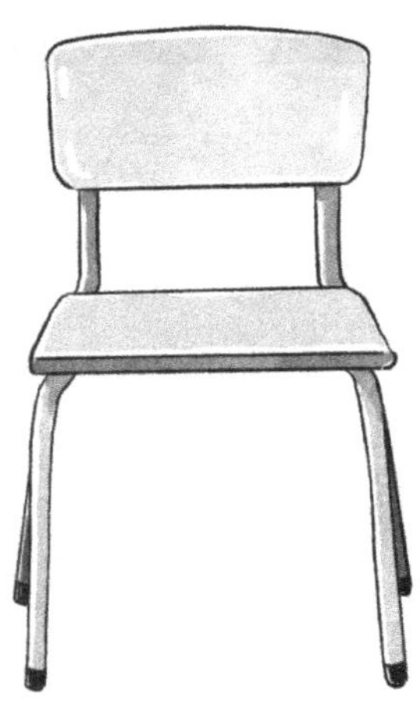

The Ultimate Manual for Boosting Strength, Stability, and Flexibility as You Age, with Effortless Daily Exercises for Seniors @ 50 and Beyond

Jerry Hargrave

THIS BOOK BELONGS TO

Disclaimer:

The information provided in this book, although fully accurate , is for informational purposes only. It is not intended to be a substitute for professional medical advice, diagnosis, or treatment. Always seek the advice of your physician or other qualified health provider with any questions you may have regarding a medical condition. Never disregard professional medical advice or delay in seeking it because of something you have read in this book.

The publisher and author are not responsible for any injuries or damages arising from the use of the information contained in this book. Readers assume full responsibility for their own health and well-being.

CONTENTS

Introduction

Welcome to "Chair Yoga for Men Over 50"!

In today's fast-paced world, finding moments of peace and tranquillity can seem like a luxury. As we get older, our bodies change, and the demands of daily life can leave us feeling stiff, achy, and out of balance. However, amidst the hustle and bustle, there is a simple yet powerful practice that provides a sanctuary—a space where we can pause, breathe, and reconnect with ourselves. That practice is known as chair yoga.

In this book, we've curated a collection of gentle but effective chair yoga exercises for men over 50. Whether you're an experienced yogi or new to the practice, you'll find simple sequences and step-by-step instructions to help you improve flexibility, strength, and inner peace.

Chair yoga isn't about twisting your body into impossible positions or pushing yourself to the limit. It's about meeting yourself right where you are, respecting your individual journey, and moving with mindful awareness. With each breath and movement, you'll learn to listen to your body, nourish your spirit, and tap into your inner wisdom.

As you embark on this journey of self-discovery and self-care, keep in mind that what matters most is the intention and presence you bring to your practice, not how perfectly you perform each pose. Allow yourself to let go of expectations, live in the present moment, and enjoy the sensations of each breath and movement.

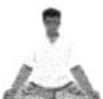

Throughout these pages, you'll discover:

- Simple yet effective exercises to relieve tension and improve mobility in key areas such as the neck, shoulders, back, hips, knees, ankles, and feet.
- Breathwork techniques to calm the mind, reduce stress, and enhance overall well-being.
- Standing poses with the support of a chair to build strength, stability, and balance.
- Practical tips and guidance for integrating chair yoga into your daily routine, no matter how busy your schedule may be.

I encourage you to use this book as a guide on your journey to better health, vitality, and joy. May it serve as a reminder that you are never too old, too stiff, or too busy to enjoy the benefits of yoga. With an open heart and a curious mind, you'll discover that the true power of chair yoga is not in what you can do, but in who you become along the way.

Namaste,

Jerry Hargrave

Chapter 1

Understanding Chair Yoga

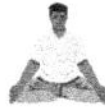

What is Chair Yoga ?

Chair yoga is a gentle form of yoga practice that is specifically designed for individuals who may have difficulty with traditional yoga poses due to mobility issues, age-related limitations, or other physical challenges. In chair yoga, practitioners perform modified yoga poses while seated on a chair or using a chair for support, making it accessible to a wide range of people, including seniors, individuals with disabilities, and those recovering from injury.

Origins and Evolution:
The roots of chair yoga can be traced back to traditional hatha yoga, which originated in ancient India thousands of years ago. Over time, yoga practitioners and instructors have adapted traditional yoga poses and techniques to accommodate the needs and abilities of diverse populations. Chair yoga has evolved as a result of these adaptations, with teachers incorporating modifications and variations to make yoga accessible to individuals who may not be able to participate in standing or floor-based yoga practices.

Principles and Practices:
Chair yoga follows the same principles as traditional yoga, including breath awareness, mindfulness, and gentle movement. Practitioners engage in a series of seated stretches, gentle twists, and mindful breathing exercises designed to improve flexibility, strength, balance, and relaxation. While seated on a chair, participants focus on connecting breath with movement, cultivating a sense of inner calm, and promoting overall well-being.

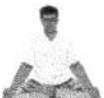

Accessibility and Inclusivity:

One of the key benefits of chair yoga is its accessibility and inclusivity. By utilizing a chair for support, individuals with limited mobility, balance issues, or chronic pain can participate in yoga practice without the need to get up and down from the floor or perform challenging standing poses. Chair yoga classes are often offered in community centers, senior centers, rehabilitation facilities, and assisted living facilities, providing a welcoming environment for individuals of all ages and abilities.

Benefits for Mind and Body:

Chair yoga offers a wide range of benefits for both the mind and body. Physically, it helps improve flexibility, mobility, and range of motion in the joints, which can alleviate stiffness and discomfort associated with conditions such as arthritis or osteoporosis. Chair yoga also strengthens the muscles, particularly in the core, legs, and arms, enhancing stability and balance. Additionally, the gentle movements and deep breathing techniques practiced in chair yoga promote relaxation, reduce stress and anxiety, and improve mental clarity and focus.

Integration with Daily Life:

One of the unique aspects of chair yoga is its integration with daily life. The principles and practices learned in chair yoga can be applied to everyday activities, such as sitting at a desk, driving a car, or performing household chores. By incorporating mindfulness, breath awareness, and gentle movement into daily routines, individuals can enhance their overall well-being and quality of life.

In summary, chair yoga offers a gentle and accessible approach to yoga practice, making it suitable for individuals of all ages and abilities.

Benefits of Chair Yoga for Seniors

1. Improved Flexibility and Range of Motion:
Chair yoga incorporates gentle stretches and movements that help seniors increase flexibility and enhance range of motion in their joints. Regular practice can alleviate stiffness, reduce discomfort, and enhance overall mobility, making daily activities easier and more comfortable.

2. Enhanced Strength and Stability:
Performing yoga poses while seated on a chair helps seniors strengthen muscles, particularly in the core, legs, and arms. This increased strength contributes to better stability and balance, reducing the risk of falls and enhancing overall functional independence.

3. Reduced Stress and Anxiety:
Chair yoga includes relaxation techniques such as deep breathing, guided imagery, and meditation, which can promote a sense of calmness and reduce stress and anxiety levels. Seniors who practice chair yoga regularly may experience improved mental well-being and greater resilience to life's challenges.

4. Improved Posture and Alignment:
Chair yoga encourages seniors to focus on proper posture and body alignment during poses and movements. This emphasis on alignment can help alleviate back pain, neck tension, and other musculoskeletal issues associated with poor posture, leading to greater comfort and ease of movement.

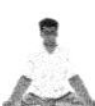

5. Enhanced Circulation and Cardiovascular Health:
The gentle movements and deep breathing exercises in chair yoga can improve blood circulation and enhance cardiovascular health. Better circulation helps deliver oxygen and nutrients to the body's tissues, promoting healing and overall vitality.

6. Boosted Mood and Emotional Well-being:
Chair yoga practice stimulates the release of endorphins, the body's natural feel-good hormones, which can uplift mood and promote a sense of well-being. Seniors may experience greater emotional resilience, improved self-esteem, and a more positive outlook on life as a result of regular chair yoga practice.

7. Social Connection and Community Engagement:
Participating in chair yoga classes provides seniors with an opportunity to connect with others in a supportive and welcoming environment. Building relationships and sharing experiences with fellow participants can combat feelings of isolation and loneliness, contributing to overall social and emotional health.

8. Adaptability and Accessibility:
Chair yoga can be easily modified to accommodate seniors of all abilities and fitness levels. Whether recovering from injury, managing chronic health conditions, or dealing with age-related limitations, seniors can tailor their practice to suit their individual needs and preferences, ensuring a safe and enjoyable yoga experience.

Getting Started with Chair Yoga

1. Set Up Your Space:

Find a quiet and comfortable area in your home where you can practice chair yoga without distractions.

Choose a sturdy chair without wheels that allows you to sit with your feet flat on the ground and your knees at a 90-degree angle.

2. Wear Comfortable Clothing:

Dress in loose, breathable clothing that allows for ease of movement.

Avoid wearing tight or restrictive clothing that may impede your ability to stretch and move comfortably.

3. Warm-Up and Center Yourself:

Begin your practice with a few minutes of deep breathing to center yourself and prepare for the session.

Sit comfortably on the chair with your feet flat on the ground and your hands resting on your thighs.

Close your eyes and take several slow, deep breaths, inhaling through your nose and exhaling through your mouth.

4. Start with Gentle Stretches:

Begin your chair yoga practice with gentle stretches to warm up your muscles and joints.

Focus on areas of tension or tightness, such as the neck, shoulders, back, and hips.

Perform simple movements such as neck rolls, shoulder shrugs, and gentle twists to loosen up your body and increase flexibility.

5. Follow a Guided Routine:

Utilize instructional videos, books, or online resources that provide chair yoga routines specifically designed for beginners.

Follow along with the instructions, paying attention to proper alignment and breathing techniques.

Start with basic poses and gradually progress to more challenging poses as you become more comfortable and confident.

6. Focus on Breath Awareness:

Incorporate mindful breathing into your chair yoga practice to enhance relaxation and reduce stress.

Coordinate your breath with movement, inhaling as you lengthen or stretch and exhaling as you release tension.

Practice deep, diaphragmatic breathing to calm the nervous system and promote a sense of inner peace.

8. End with Relaxation and Meditation:

Conclude your chair yoga practice with a few minutes of relaxation and meditation.

Sit comfortably on the chair with your eyes closed and your hands resting on your lap.

Take slow, deep breaths, allowing your body to relax completely and your mind to quieten.

Visualize a peaceful scene or repeat a calming mantra to promote relaxation and mental clarity.

9. Reflect and Rejuvenate:

Take a moment to reflect on how you feel after your chair yoga practice. Notice any changes in your body, mind, or mood, and acknowledge the benefits of your practice.

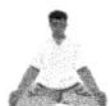

Equipments

1. Sturdy Chair:

Choose a sturdy chair without wheels, preferably with a straight back and no armrests.

Ensure the chair is placed on a stable surface to prevent slipping during practice.

2. Yoga Blocks:

Yoga blocks can be used to provide additional support and stability during certain poses.

They can be placed under the feet, hands, or hips tc modify poses and accommodate individual needs.

3. Yoga Strap:

A yoga strap can help increase flexibility and improve alignment by extending your reach in certain poses.

Use the strap to gently stretch tight muscles or to maintain proper alignment in seated or reclining poses.

4. Yoga Blanket or Towel:

A yoga blanket or towel can provide cushioning and support during seated poses and relaxation exercises.

Fold the blanket or towel to create additional padding for your seat or to support your knees and ankles.

5. Water Bottle:

Stay hydrated during your chair yoga practice by keeping a water bottle nearby.

Take sips of water as needed to replenish fluids and stay energized throughout your practice.

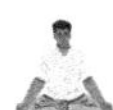

6. Comfortable Clothing:

Wear loose, comfortable clothing that allows for ease of movement and flexibility.

Choose breathable fabrics that wick away moisture and keep you comfortable during your practice.

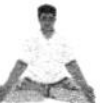

Chapter 2

Basic Chair Yoga Poses

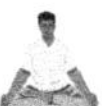

Seated Cat-Cow Stretch

- Begin by sitting comfortably in a chair, feet flat on the floor, hands resting on your knees.
- As you inhale, gently arch your back, lifting your chest to the ceiling and drawing your shoulder blades together. This is the Cow part of the stretch.
- Exhale by rounding your spine, tucking your chin against your chest, and drawing your navel towards your spine. Feel a stretch in your upper back. This is the Cat section of the stretch.
- Repeat this movement several times, alternating between Cow and Cat with each breath, allowing the movement to be fluid and gentle.
- Concentrate on matching your breath to the movement, inhaling as you arch into Cow and exhaling as you round into Cat.
- Continue to take as many breaths as you feel comfortable, allowing your spine to gently warm up and release tension.

Reflection Box

Short description of how you felt during the pose and how you want to improve next time

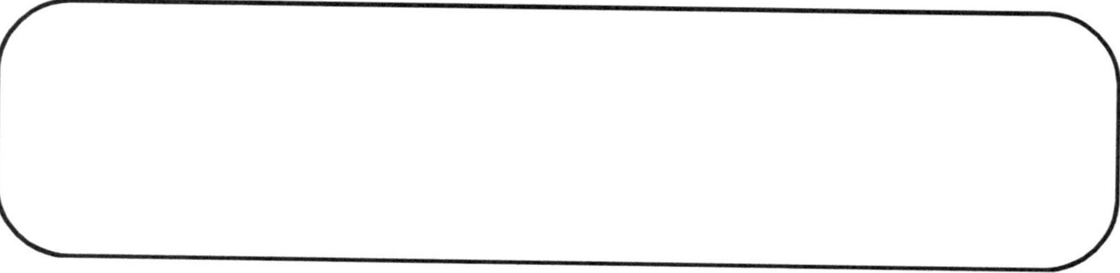

Seated Spinal Twist

- Sit at the front edge of your chair, feet flat on the floor, spine tall.
- Place your left hand on the outside of your right knee or thigh, and your right hand on the chair's backrest or seat for support.
- Inhale to lengthen your spine, and as you exhale, gently twist to the right, using your hands to deepen the twist as needed.
- Turn your head to look over your right shoulder while keeping your spine length and both sit bones firmly planted in the chair.
- Hold the twist for a few breaths, feeling the gentle stretch along the spine and torso.
- On an inhale, slowly release the twist and turn to face forward.
- Repeat the twist on the opposite side, with your right hand on the outside of your left knee or thigh and your left hand providing support.
- Hold the twist for a few breaths while remaining aware of your breathing and body sensations.

Reflection Box

Short description of how you felt during the pose and how you want to improve next time

Seated Forward Fold

- Sit at the front edge of your chair, feet hip-width apart and spine tall.
- Inhale to lengthen your spine, then exhale, hinge forward from your hips while keeping your back straight.
- Lower your chest towards your thighs, allowing your hands to hang down to the floor or hold onto the chair's legs for support.
- Relax your neck and shoulders, allowing your head to hang heavy on the floor.
- Take several deep breaths while in this position, feeling the stretch in your spine, hamstrings, and lower back.
- On an inhale, slowly rise back to a seated position, stacking your vertebrae one at a time.
- Repeat the forward fold several times, moving with your breath and responding to your body's cues.

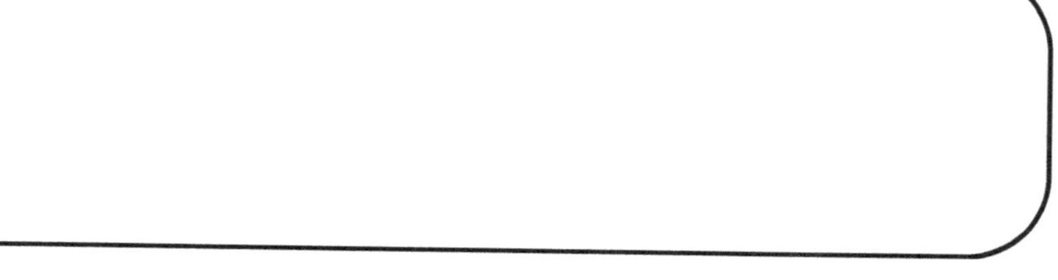

Reflection Box

Short description of how you felt during the pose and how you want to improve next time

Seated Mountain Pose

- Sit tall in your chair, feet flat on the floor, hands resting on your thighs.
- Ground down through your sit bones, feeling stable and supported by the chair beneath you.
- Inhale and lengthen your spine, lifting through the crown of your head to the ceiling.
- Exhale as you engage your core muscles and gently draw your navel towards your spine.
- Reach your arms overhead, palms facing each other, and actively press your hands toward the ceiling to feel a stretch in your sides and arms.
- Hold the pose for a few breaths, feeling grounded in your lower body and reaching energetically with your fingertips.
- On an exhale, lower your arms to your sides and return to a neutral seated position.
- Repeat the pose several times, focusing on the relationship between breath, movement, and alignment.

Reflection Box

Short description of how you felt during the pose and how you want to improve next time

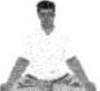

Seated Shoulder Rolls

- Sit comfortably in your chair, feet flat on the floor, hands resting on your thighs.
- Inhale as you raise your shoulders to your ears, squeezing them up towards the ceiling.
- Exhale while rolling your shoulders back and down, bringing your shoulder blades together and expanding your chest.
- Continue to roll your shoulders in smooth circles, forward, up, backward, and down.
- With each roll, work to relieve tension and tightness in the shoulders and upper back.
- After a few rounds in one direction, switch directions and roll your shoulders the opposite way.
- Continue to move with your breath, taking your time to find any areas of tightness or restriction in your shoulders.
- When you're finished, pause and allow your shoulders to relax away from your ears.

Reflection Box

Short description of how you felt during the pose and how you want to improve next time

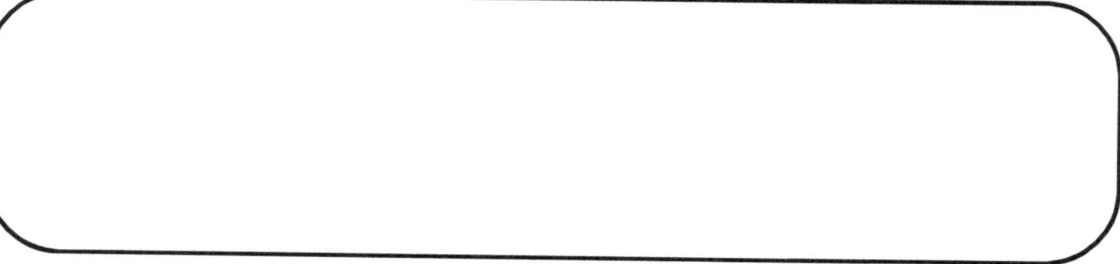

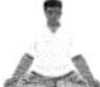

Chapter 3

Breathe

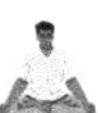

Deep Belly Breathing

- Find a comfortable seated position, either in a chair with your feet flat on the floor or on the ground, legs crossed.
- Place your hands gently on your abdomen, just below the ribcage.
- Close your eyes and take a few natural breaths, noting how your belly rises and falls with each inhale and exhale.
- Begin inhaling deeply through your nose, allowing your belly to fill completely with air. Feel your hands rise as your abdomen expands with breath.
- Exhale slowly and completely through your nose, allowing your belly to gently contract as you release the breath.
- Continue this deep belly breathing pattern for a few minutes, focusing on the sensation of your breath moving in and out of your body, as well as the rhythmic rise and fall of your abdomen.

Reflection Box

Short description of how you felt during the pose and how you want to improve next time

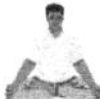

4-7-8 Breath

- Sit comfortably with your back straight, either in a chair with your feet flat on the floor or on the ground, legs crossed.
- Place the tip of your tongue against the ridge of tissue just behind your upper front teeth and hold there throughout the exercise.
- Close your mouth and inhale quietly through your nose for four seconds.
- Hold your breath for seven seconds.
- Exhale completely through your mouth, making a whooshing sound for a count of eight seconds.
- Repeat this cycle for four breaths, relaxing deeper with each exhalation.

Reflection Box

Short description of how you felt during the pose and how you want to improve next time

Alternate Nostril Breathing

- Sit comfortably in a chair, back straight, or cross-legged on the floor.
- Rest your left hand on your left knee, palm facing upward.
- Close your right nostril gently with your right thumb and take a deep breath in through your left.
- Close your left nostril with your right ring finger, then remove your thumb from your right nostril.
- Exhale completely through your right nostril.
- Inhale deeply through your right nostril.
- Close your right nostril with your right thumb while releasing your left nostril.
- Exhale completely through the left nostril.
- This concludes one round of alternate nostril breathing. Repeat several times, beginning and ending with an inhalation through the left nostril.

Reflection Box

Short description of how you felt during the pose and how you want to improve next time

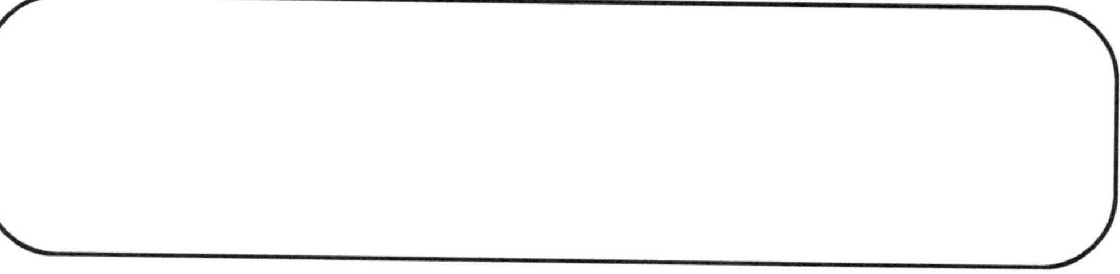

Ocean Breathing (Ujjayi Pranayama)

- Sit comfortably in a chair or on the floor, keeping your spine tall and your shoulders relaxed.
- Inhale deeply through your nose, filling your lungs entirely.
- Exhale through your mouth, making a soft "ha" sound as if you were fogging up a mirror.
- Now close your mouth and exhale through your nose, making the same "ha" sound but with your mouth closed.
- Continue to breathe rhythmically, feeling the slight constriction in the back of your throat that produces the ocean-like sound.
- Match the length and intensity of each inhale and exhale, resulting in a smooth and consistent flow of breath.

Reflection Box

Short description of how you felt during the pose and how you want to improve next time

Three-Part Breath (Dirga Pranayama)

- Find a comfortable seated position, either in a chair with your feet flat on the floor or on the ground, legs crossed.
- Place your hands on your abdomen, just beneath your ribs.
- Close your eyes and take a few natural breaths, noting how your belly rises and falls with each inhale and exhale.
- Begin by inhaling deeply through your nose, allowing your belly to completely expand with air. Feel your hands rise as your abdomen expands with breath.
- Continue inhaling, allowing the breath to fill your ribcage and expand your chest completely.
- Finally, inhale deeply into your upper chest, feeling your collarbones lift slightly as you fill the uppermost part of your lungs with oxygen.
- Exhale slowly and completely, allowing the breath to leave your chest, ribs, and abdomen in a smooth and controlled manner.
- Repeat this three-part breath pattern several times, focusing on how your breath moves through each part of your body, creating a sense of expansion and relaxation.

Reflection Box

Short description of how you felt during the pose and how you want to improve next time

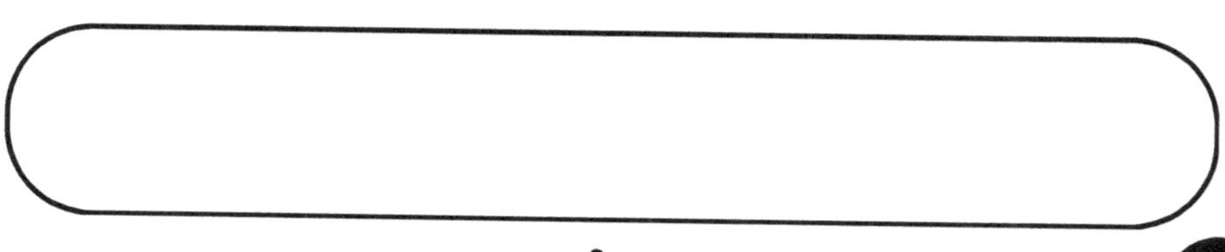

Chapter 4

Warm Up

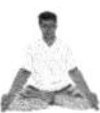

Seated Side Stretch

- Sit comfortably in a chair, feet flat on the floor and spine upright.
- Stretch your right arm overhead, towards the left side.
- Inhale deeply to lengthen your spine, and as you exhale, lean to the left while keeping both hips grounded in the chair.
- Feel the stretch on the right side of your body, from your fingertips to your hip.
- Hold the stretch for a few breaths and feel a gentle opening in your side body.
- Inhale to return to center, then repeat on the opposite side, raising your left arm overhead and leaning to the right.

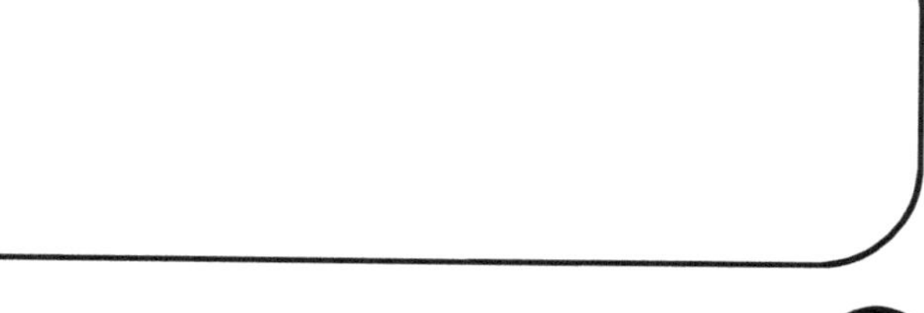

Reflection Box

Short description of how you felt during the pose and how you want to improve next time

Seated Twist With Arm Reach

- Sit comfortably in a chair, feet flat on the floor and spine upright.
- Inhale to lengthen your spine, then exhale, twisting your torso to the right.
- Place your left hand on the outside of your right knee or thigh to provide support.
- Reach your right arm behind you and rest your hand on the backrest or seat of the chair.
- Inhale to lengthen your spine further, and then exhale to deepen the twist by gently looking over your right shoulder.
- Hold the twist for a few breaths to feel the stretch in your spine and shoulders.
- Inhale to return to center, then repeat the twist on the opposite side, twisting to the left and reaching your left arm back.

Reflection Box

Short description of how you felt during the pose and how you want to improve next time

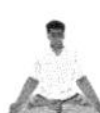

Neck Rolls

- Sit comfortably in a chair, feet flat on the floor and spine upright.
- Drop your chin to your chest and feel a gentle stretch along the back of your neck.
- Slowly roll your head to the right, bringing your right ear near your right shoulder.
- Continue to roll your head back, bringing your chin to the ceiling, and then to the left, bringing your left ear to your left shoulder.
- Complete the circle by bringing your chin back to your chest.
- Repeat this circular motion in the opposite direction, beginning with a left roll of the head.
- Move slowly and mindfully, pausing at any points of tension to breathe deeply and relieve tension.

Reflection Box

Short description of how you felt during the pose and how you want to improve next time

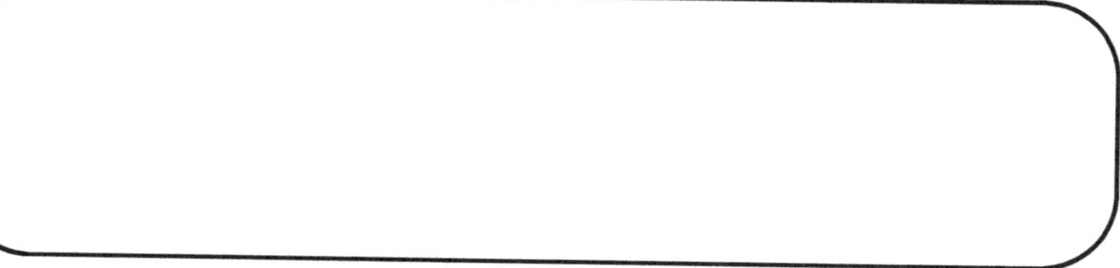

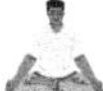

Shoulder Circles

- Sit comfortably in a chair, feet flat on the floor and spine upright.
- Inhale as you raise your shoulders to your ears, squeezing them up towards the ceiling.
- Exhale while rolling your shoulders back and down, bringing your shoulder blades together and expanding your chest.
- Continue rolling your shoulders in smooth circles, forward, up, back, and down.
- With each roll, work to relieve tension and tightness in the shoulders and upper back.
- After a few rounds in one direction, switch directions and roll your shoulders the opposite way.
- Continue to move with your breath, taking your time to find any areas of tightness or restriction in your shoulders.

Reflection Box

Short description of how you felt during the pose and how you want to improve next time

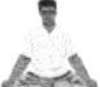

Wrist Circles

- Sit comfortably in a chair, feet flat on the floor and spine upright.
- Extend your arms out in front of you to shoulder height, palms facing down.
- Begin to move your wrists in small circles clockwise.
- Concentrate on moving from the wrists while keeping your arms and shoulders relaxed.
- After a few rotations, switch to counterclockwise circles and move in the opposite direction.
- Continue to move with your breath, pausing to investigate any areas of tension or discomfort in the wrists.
- After making several circles in each direction, shake your hands and wrists to relieve any remaining tension.

Reflection Box

Short description of how you felt during the pose and how you want to improve next time

Chapter 5

Balance

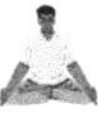

Seated Knee Lifts

- Sit comfortably in a chair, feet flat on the floor and spine upright.
- Place your hands on the chair's sides to provide support.
- Inhale deeply and engage your core muscles.
- Exhale as you lift your right knee to your chest while keeping your foot flexed.
- Hold the lifted position for a moment, feeling the abdominal muscles engage and the hip flexors stretch.
- Inhale and lower your right foot back to the ground.
- Repeat the movement on the left side, raising your left knee to your chest.
- Continue alternating between lifting each knee for several repetitions, moving with your breath and maintaining proper posture.

Reflection Box

Short description of how you felt during the pose and how you want to improve next time

Seated Leg Extensions

- Sit comfortably in a chair, feet flat on the floor and spine upright.
- Hold onto the chair's sides for support.
- Prepare by inhaling deeply.
- Exhale and extend your right leg straight out in front of you, engaging your quadriceps.
- Point your toes towards the ceiling and feel a stretch in the back of your leg.
- Hold the extended position for a moment, then inhale to bend your right knee and lower your foot to the floor.
- Repeat the movement on the left side, extending your left leg straight ahead of you.
- Continue to alternate between extending each leg for several repetitions, moving with your breath and maintaining proper posture.

Reflection Box

Short description of how you felt during the pose and how you want to improve next time

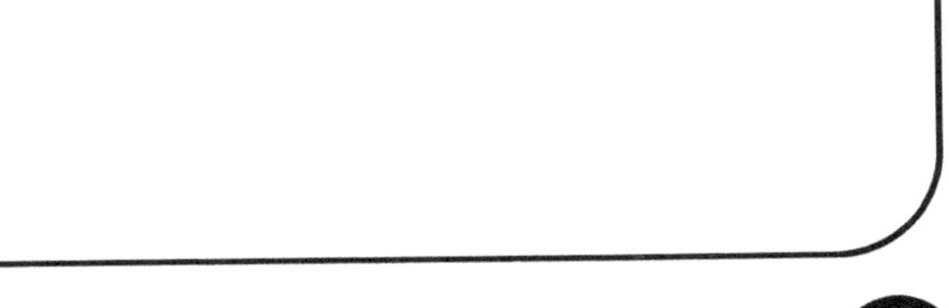

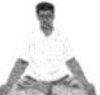

Seated Figure Four Stretch

- Sit comfortably in a chair, feet flat on the floor and spine upright.
- Cross your right ankle over your left knee, and flex your right foot to protect your knee joint.
- Keep your right knee pointing to the side.
- Inhale deeply to lengthen your spine.
- Exhale while gently pressing down on your right knee with your right hand, causing a stretch in your outer right hip.
- Hold the stretch for a few breaths, letting your muscles relax and release.
- Inhale to relieve pressure on your knee; exhale to uncross your right leg and return to the starting position.
- Repeat the stretch on the opposite side, crossing your left ankle over your right knee.

Reflection Box

Short description of how you felt during the pose and how you want to improve next time

Seated Tree Pose

- Sit comfortably in a chair, feet flat on the floor and spine upright.
- Use your core muscles to stabilize your pelvis.
- Inhale deeply to lengthen your spine.
- Exhale as you lift your right foot off the ground, placing the sole of your right foot against the inside of your left leg.
- Press your right foot firmly into your left thigh, then your left thigh into your right foot, resulting in gentle resistance.
- Bring your hands to your heart center in a prayer position, or extend them overhead for an extra stretch.
- Hold the pose for a few breaths to find your balance and focus.
- Inhale to release the pose, then exhale to return your right foot to the ground.
- Repeat the pose on the opposite side, lifting your left foot and placing it against the inside of your right thigh.

Reflection Box

Short description of how you felt during the pose and how you want to improve next time

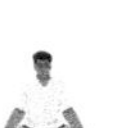

Seated Eagle Arms

- Sit comfortably in a chair, feet flat on the floor and spine upright.
- Extend your arms out to the sides, shoulder height.
- Cross your right arm over your left, bringing the palms together if possible.
- If your palms do not meet, you can bring the backs of your hands together or simply hug yourself, placing your hands on opposite shoulders.
- Lift your elbows slightly and feel the stretch between your shoulder blades.
- Hold the pose for a few moments, taking deep breaths into the stretch.
- Inhale to release the pose, then exhale to extend your arms out to the sides.
- Repeat the pose but this time cross your left arm over your right.

Reflection Box

Short description of how you felt during the pose and how you want to improve next time

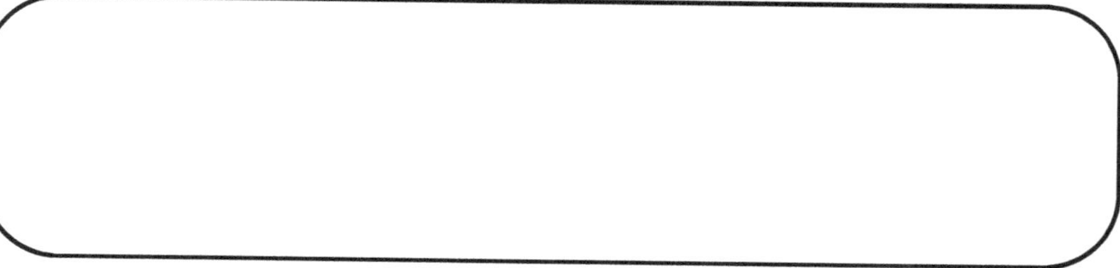

Chapter 6

Neck and Shoulders

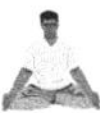

Neck Side Stretch

- Sit comfortably in a chair, feet flat on the floor and spine upright.
- Relax your shoulders down and away from your ears.
- Inhale deeply, lengthening your spine.
- As you exhale, tilt your head to the right, bringing your right ear close to your right shoulder.
- Keep your shoulders relaxed and refrain from lifting or rounding them.
- Hold the stretch for 15-30 seconds to feel a gentle stretch along the left side of your neck.
- Inhale to return to center, then exhale as you tilt your head to the left, bringing your left ear near your left shoulder.
- Hold the stretch for 15-30 seconds to feel a gentle stretch along the right side of your neck.
- Repeat on both sides 2-3 times, taking deep breaths and relaxing into the stretch.

Reflection Box

Short description of how you felt during the pose and how you want to improve next time

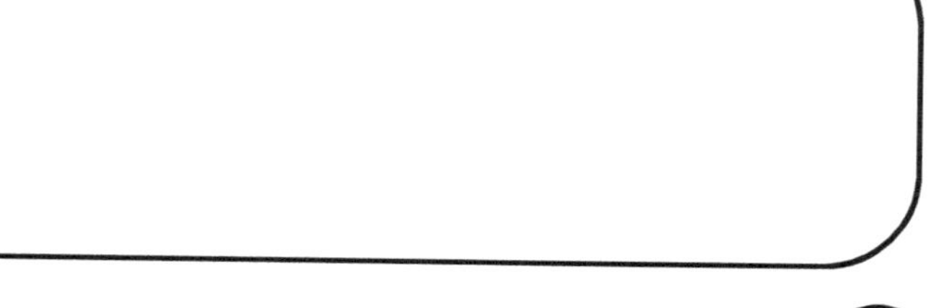

Shoulder Shrug and Release

- Sit comfortably in a chair, feet flat on the floor and spine upright.
- Relax your arms at your sides and, if comfortable, close your eyes.
- Inhale deeply through your nose.
- As you exhale, shrug your shoulders up towards your ears, causing tension in your shoulders.
- Hold the shrug for a moment and feel the tension in your shoulders.
- Inhale deeply again.
- As you exhale, lower your shoulders and let go of any tension.
- Allow your shoulders to naturally drop, resulting in a sense of relaxation and relief.
- Repeat the shoulder shrug and release exercise 2-3 times, moving with your breath and concentrating on releasing tension with each exhale.

Reflection Box

Short description of how you felt during the pose and how you want to improve next time

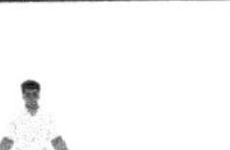

Seated Shoulder Opener

- Sit comfortably in a chair, feet flat on the floor and spine upright.
- Reach your arms behind you and grab the back of the chair with your hands.
- Inhale deeply, lengthening your spine.
- As you exhale, gently press your chest forward and raise your chin to the ceiling.
- Maintain a relaxed shoulder posture and avoid hunching or rounding.
- Hold the stretch for 15 to 30 seconds, feeling a gentle opening in your chest and shoulders.
- Inhale to return to the center, then exhale as you relax the stretch.
- Repeat the shoulder opener 2-3 times, breathing deeply while relaxing into the stretch.

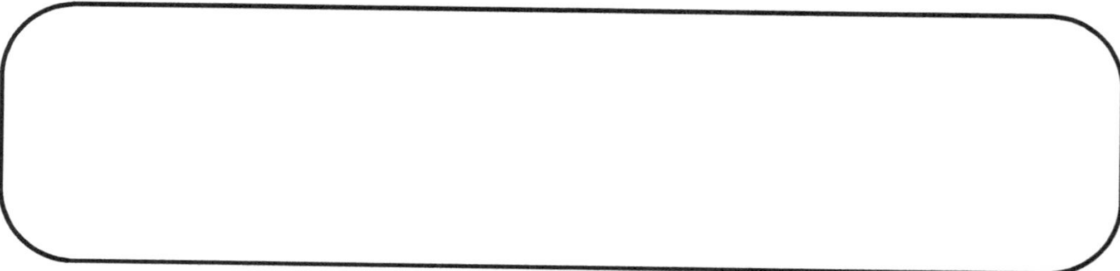

Reflection Box

Short description of how you felt during the pose and how you want to improve next time

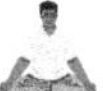

Neck Circles

- Sit comfortably in a chair, feet flat on the floor and spine upright.
- Relax your shoulders down and away from your ears.
- Inhale deeply to lengthen your spine.
- As you exhale, gently lower your chin to your chest, feeling a stretch in the back of your neck.
- Slowly circle your head to the right, first bringing your right ear to your right shoulder, then lifting your chin to the ceiling, and finally bringing your left ear to your left shoulder.
- Continue to circle your head in this direction 4-5 times, moving slowly and deliberately.
- Then, reverse the direction of the circles, beginning with your left ear and moving to your left shoulder.
- Circle your head to the left, raising your chin to the ceiling and then bringing your right ear to your right shoulder.
- Continue to circle your head in this direction 4-5 times, moving with your breath and concentrating on relaxing your neck.

Reflection Box

Short description of how you felt during the pose and how you want to improve next time

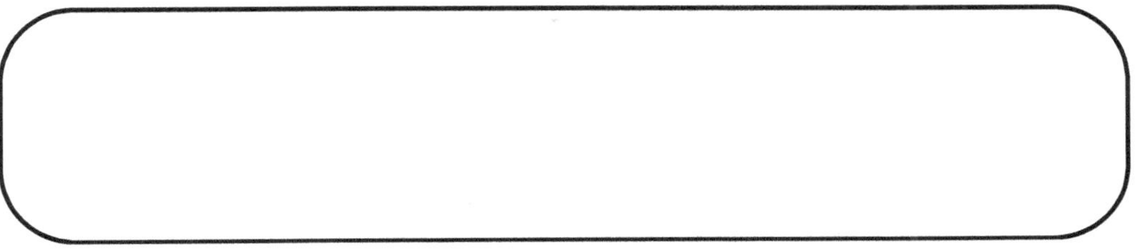

"

Seated Shoulder Stretch

- Sit comfortably in a chair, feet flat on the floor and spine upright.
- Reach your right arm across your chest, keeping it straight, and rest your left hand on your elbow.
- Pull your right arm gently towards your chest, allowing your right shoulder and upper arm muscles to stretch.
- Keep your shoulders relaxed and refrain from lifting or rounding them.
- Hold the stretch for 15 to 30 seconds, breathing deeply and concentrating on releasing tension.
- Inhale to relax the stretch, then exhale to switch sides.
- Reach your left arm across your chest, and place your right hand on your left elbow.
- Pull your left arm gently towards your chest until you feel a stretch in your left shoulder and upper arm muscles.
- Hold the stretch for 15 to 30 seconds, breathing deeply and relaxing into it.

Reflection Box

Short description of how you felt during the pose and how you want to improve next time

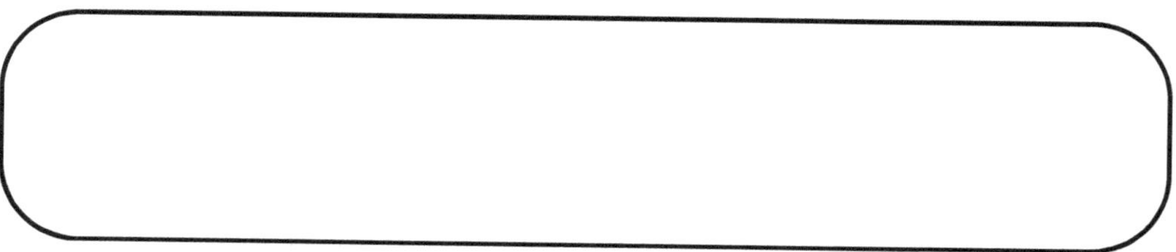

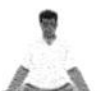

Seated Shoulder Blade Squeeze

- Sit tall in your chair, feet flat on the floor, spine comfortably upright.
- Relax your shoulders away from your ears and let your arms rest gently by your sides.
- Take a deep breath in, bringing your attention to your shoulder blades.
- As you exhale, gently squeeze your shoulder blades together, bringing them closer to your spine. Imagine trying to hold a pencil between your shoulder blades.
- Hold the squeeze for a moment, feeling the muscles between your shoulder blades engage and the front of your chest expand.
- When performing the squeeze, keep your shoulders from hunching or lifting towards your ears.
- Inhale as you let go of the squeeze, allowing your shoulder blades to gently slide apart.
- Repeat the movement several times, coordinating your breath with each squeeze and release.
- Maintain good posture and alignment throughout the exercise, with your spine tall and your chest open.

Reflection Box

Short description of how you felt during the pose and how you want to improve next time

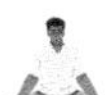

Chapter 7

Hands and Arms

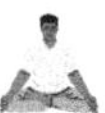

Seated Wrist Flexor Stretch

- Sit comfortably in a chair, feet flat on the floor and spine upright.
- Extend your right arm straight in front of you, palm facing down.
- Stretch your wrist and fingers by gently pressing down on your right hand's fingers with your left hand.
- Hold the stretch for 15-30 seconds to feel a gentle stretch along the underside of your right wrist and forearm.
- Release the stretch and switch sides, extending your left arm in front of you and pressing down on the fingers with your right hand.
- Hold the stretch for 15 to 30 seconds, breathing deeply and relaxing into it.

Reflection Box

Short description of how you felt during the pose and how you want to improve next time

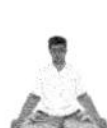

Seated Wrist Extensor Stretch

- Sit comfortably in a chair, feet flat on the floor and spine upright.
- Extend your right arm straight in front of you, palm facing up.
- Use your left hand to gently press down on the back of your right hand, stretching the wrist and fingers.
- Hold the stretch for 15-30 seconds to feel a gentle stretch along the top of your right wrist and forearm.
- Release the stretch and switch sides, extending your left arm in front of you and pressing down on the back of your hand with your right.
- Hold the stretch for 15 to 30 seconds, breathing deeply and relaxing into it.

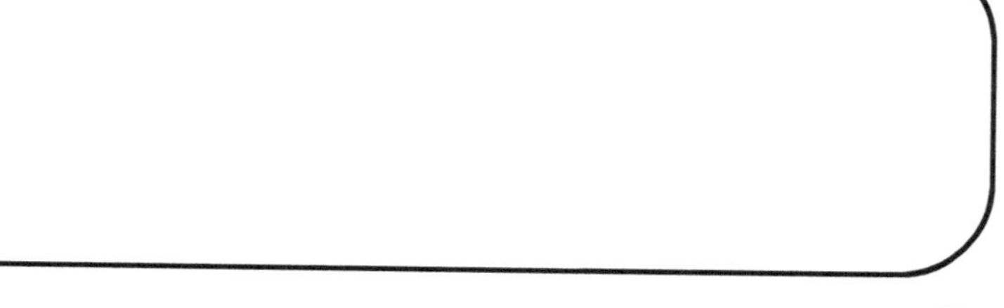

Reflection Box

Short description of how you felt during the pose and how you want to improve next time

Fist-to-Fan Stretch

- Sit comfortably in a chair, feet flat on the floor and spine upright.
- Extend both arms straight out in front of you at shoulder level, palms down.
- Make fists with both hands, curling your fingers into your palms.
- Prepare by inhaling deeply.
- Exhale and open your hands into a "fan" shape, spreading your fingers wide apart.
- Hold the stretch for a moment to feel a gentle stretch in your palms and fingers.
- Inhale to return to fists, curling your fingers into your palms.
- Exhale to reopen into a fan shape, spreading your fingers apart.
- Repeat this movement several times, moving with your breath and concentrating on the sensation of opening and stretching in your hands and fingers.

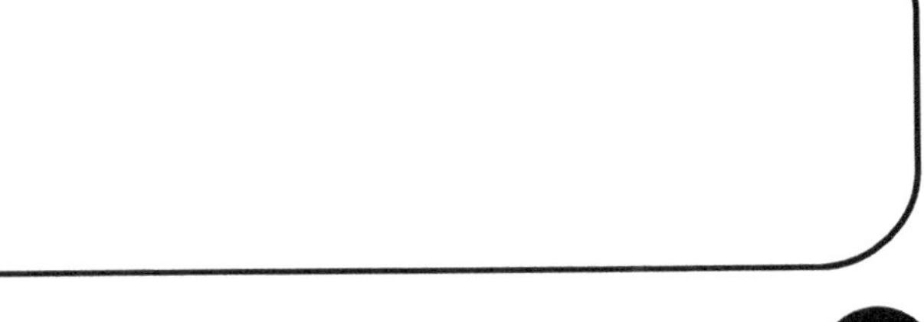

Reflection Box

Short description of how you felt during the pose and how you want to improve next time

Seated Arm Circles

- Sit comfortably in a chair, feet flat on the floor and spine upright.
- Extend both arms to the sides at shoulder height, palms facing down.
- Prepare by inhaling deeply.
- As you exhale, begin to move your arms forward in small, controlled circles.
- Continue to circle your arms forward 4-5 times, keeping your shoulders relaxed and your core engaged.
- Inhale and pause at the top of the circle.
- Exhale as you reverse the direction of the circles and circle your arms backwards.
- Continue to circle your arms backward for 4-5 rotations, moving with your breath and concentrating on smooth, controlled motion.

Reflection Box

Short description of how you felt during the pose and how you want to improve next time

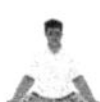

Seated Triceps Stretch

- Sit comfortably in a chair, feet flat on the floor and spine upright.
- Extend your right arm overhead, palm facing inward, to reach the ceiling.
- Bend your right elbow and bring your right hand to the middle of your upper back.
- Use your left hand to gently press down on your right elbow to increase the stretch in your right triceps.
- Maintain a relaxed shoulder posture and avoid hunching or rounding.
- Hold the stretch for 15-30 seconds to feel a gentle stretch along the back of your right arm.
- Inhale to relax the stretch, then exhale to switch sides.
- Extend your left arm overhead, bending the elbow and placing the left hand in the center of your upper back.
- Use your right hand to gently press down on your left elbow to increase the stretch in your left triceps.
- Hold the stretch for 15 to 30 seconds, breathing deeply and relaxing into it.

Reflection Box

Short description of how you felt during the pose and how you want to improve next time

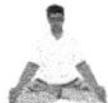

Chapter 8

Abdominals

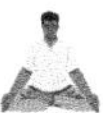

Seated Knee-to-Chest Stretch

- Sit comfortably in a chair, feet flat on the floor and spine upright.
- Inhale deeply to lengthen your spine.
- Exhale and lift your right knee to your chest, wrapping your arms around your shin or knee.
- Keep your left foot firmly on the ground.
- Hold the stretch for a few breaths until you feel a gentle compression in your hips and lower back.
- Inhale to lower your right leg to the floor.
- Repeat the stretch on the left side, bringing your left knee to your chest and holding for a few breaths.
- Continue alternating between both legs for several repetitions, moving with your breath and concentrating on the sensation of the stretch.

Reflection Box

Short description of how you felt during the pose and how you want to improve next time

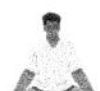

Seated Abdominal Twist

- Sit comfortably in a chair, feet flat on the floor and spine upright.
- Inhale deeply to lengthen your spine.
- Exhale as you twist your torso to the right, resting your left hand on the outside of your right knee and your right hand on the chair's back for support.
- Maintain a tall spine and relaxed shoulders as you deepen the twist.
- Inhale to lengthen your spine further, and exhale to twist slightly deeper.
- Hold the twist for a few breaths to feel a gentle stretch in your spine and abdominal muscles.
- Inhale to return to center, and then exhale as you twist to the left, resting your right hand on the outside of your left knee and your left hand on the back of the chair.
- Hold the twist on this side for a few breaths, inhaling deeply and relaxing into the stretch.

Reflection Box

Short description of how you felt during the pose and how you want to improve next time

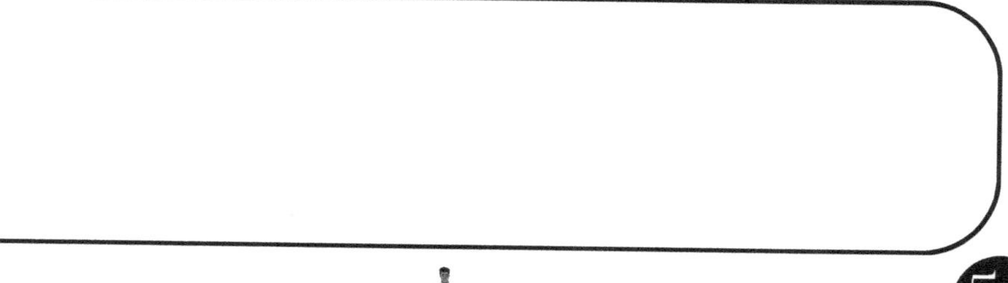

Seated Boat Pose

- Sit comfortably in a chair, feet flat on the floor and spine upright.
- Place your hands on the chair's sides to provide support.
- Inhale deeply to lengthen your spine.
- Exhale and lean back slightly, lifting your feet off the floor and straightening your legs.
- To maintain balance, engage your core muscles while keeping your spine tall and your chest lifted.
- Hold the pose for a few breaths, noticing the engagement of your abdominal muscles.
- Inhale to release the pose and return your feet to the ground.
- Repeat the pose several times, moving with your breath and concentrating on maintaining proper posture and stability.

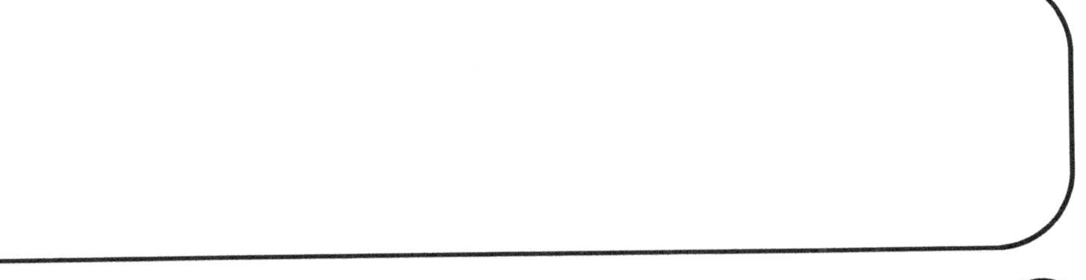

Reflection Box

Short description of how you felt during the pose and how you want to improve next time

Seated Crunches

- Sit comfortably in a chair, feet flat on the floor and spine upright.
- Place your hands behind your head, interlocking your fingers or gently supporting your head with your fingertips.
- Prepare by inhaling deeply.
- Exhale as you contract your abdominal muscles and raise your chest towards your thighs, bringing your elbows to your knees.
- Hold the crunch for a moment and feel the contraction in your abdominal muscles.
- Inhale to release the crunch, then lower your chest back into the chair.
- Repeat the crunch several times, moving with your breath and concentrating on the engagement of your core muscles.

Reflection Box

Short description of how you felt during the pose and how you want to improve next time

Seated Bicycle Crunches

- Sit comfortably in a chair, feet flat on the floor and spine upright.
- Place your hands behind your head, interlocking your fingers or gently supporting your head with your fingertips.
- Prepare by inhaling deeply.
- Exhale as you lift your right knee to your chest and rotate your torso to bring your left elbow near your right knee.
- Inhale while lowering your right leg to the floor and returning to the starting position.
- Exhale as you lift your left knee to your chest and rotate your torso to bring your right elbow near your left knee.
- Continue to alternate between right and left knee lifts, keeping a fluid and controlled motion.
- Repeat the bicycle crunches several times, moving with your breath and keeping your core muscles engaged.

Reflection Box

Short description of how you felt during the pose and how you want to improve next time

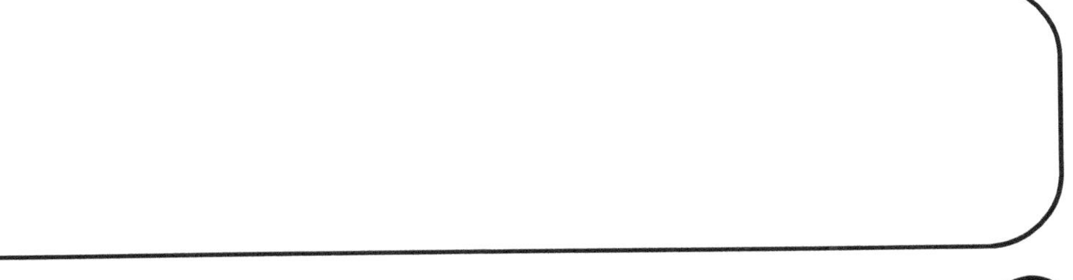

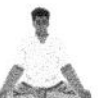

Chapter 9

Middle and Lower Back

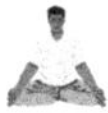

Seated Cat-Cow Stretch

- Sit comfortably in a chair, feet flat on the floor and spine upright.
- Put your hands on your knees or thighs.
- Inhale deeply, arch your back, lift your chest, and bring your shoulder blades together in Cow Pose.
- Exhale and round your spine, tucking your chin to your chest and bringing your belly button close to your spine (Cat Pose).
- Flow smoothly between Cow and Cat poses, following your breath.
- Repeat for several rounds, paying special attention to spine movement as well as chest and abdomen expansion and contraction.

Reflection Box

Short description of how you felt during the pose and how you want to improve next time

Seated Spinal Twist

- Sit comfortably in a chair, feet flat on the floor and spine upright.
- Inhale to lengthen the spine.
- Exhale while twisting your torso to the right, with your left hand on your right knee and your right hand on the back of the chair.
- Maintain a tall spine and relaxed shoulders as you deepen the twist.
- Inhale to lengthen your spine further, and exhale to twist slightly deeper.
- Hold the twist for a few breaths, feeling a gentle stretch along your spine and torso.
- Inhale to return to center, and then exhale as you twist to the left, resting your right hand on your left knee and your left hand on the back of the chair.
- Hold the twist on this side for a few breaths, inhaling deeply and relaxing into the stretch.

Reflection Box

Short description of how you felt during the pose and how you want to improve next time

Seated Forward Fold

- Sit at the front edge of a chair, your feet hip-width apart and your spine upright.
- Inhale deeply to lengthen your spine.
- Exhale as you hinge forward from your hips, bringing your hands to your feet or the floor.
- Keep your back straight and fold forward, leading with your chest.
- Allow your head to fall towards your knees, feeling a stretch along the spine and down the backs of your legs.
- Hold the forward fold for a few breaths before relaxing into the stretch.
- Inhale and slowly lift yourself back up to a seated position, stacking your vertebrae one by one

Reflection Box

Short description of how you felt during the pose and how you want to improve next time

Seated Child Pose

- Sit comfortably in a chair, knees bent, feet flat on the floor.
- Separate your knees slightly more than hip width apart.
- Inhale deeply to lengthen your spine.
- Exhale as you hinge forward from your hips and lower your chest to your thighs.
- Allow your forehead to rest on the chair's seat or a block placed between your legs.
- Extend your arms forward on the chair's seat or the floor, bringing your fingertips away from your body.
- Relax your shoulders and neck, then breathe deeply into your back body.
- Hold the pose for a few breaths to feel a gentle stretch in your hips, lower back, and spine.
- To exit the pose, inhale as you raise your torso back to a sitting position.

Reflection Box

Short description of how you felt during the pose and how you want to improve next time

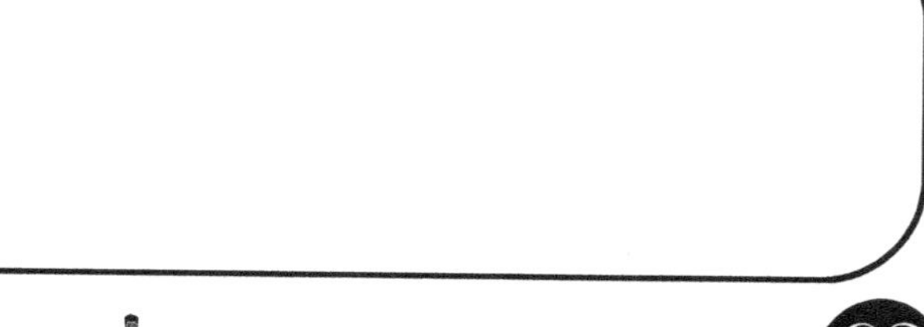

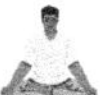

Seated Pelvic Tilts

- Sit comfortably in a chair, feet flat on the floor and spine upright.
- Put your hands on your hips for support.
- Inhale deeply to lengthen your spine.
- Exhale by tilting your pelvis forward, arching your lower back, and extending your tailbone behind you.
- Hold the tilt for a moment to feel a stretch in the front of your hips and abdomen.
- Inhale to return to the neutral pelvis position.
- Exhale by tilting your pelvis backward, rounding your lower back, and tucking your tailbone under.
- Hold the tilt for a moment to feel a stretch in the back of your hips and lower back.
- Continue to alternate between forward and backward pelvic tilts, following your breath and focusing on the movement of your pelvis.

Reflection Box

Short description of how you felt during the pose and how you want to improve next time

Chapter 10

Hips

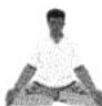

Seated Hip Flexor Stretch

- Sit comfortably in a chair, feet flat on the floor and spine upright.
- Slide your right foot back slightly, then extend your right leg behind you.
- Keep your right knee bent and your toes pointing down to the floor.
- Inhale deeply to lengthen your spine.
- Exhale and gently lean forward, feeling a stretch in the front of your right hip and thigh.
- Keep your left foot flat on the ground and your left knee directly above your left ankle.
- Hold the stretch for 15 to 30 seconds, breathing deeply and relaxing into it.
- Inhale to relax the stretch, then exhale while switching sides, sliding your left foot back and stretching your left hip flexor.

Reflection Box

Short description of how you felt during the pose and how you want to improve next time

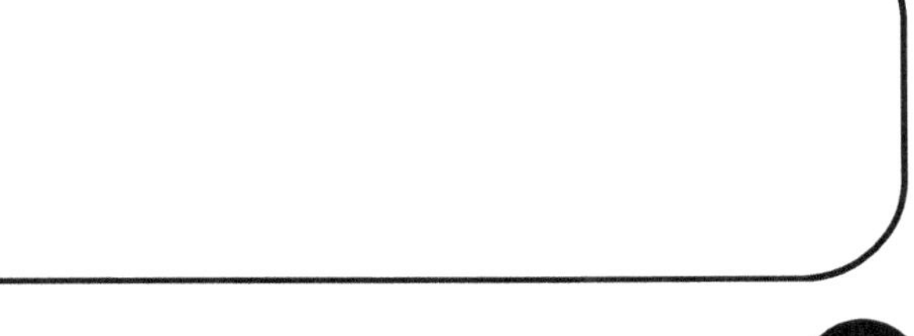

Seated Pigeon Pose

- Sit comfortably in a chair, feet flat on the floor and spine upright.
- Lift your right foot off the floor, then place your right ankle on top of your left thigh, just above your knee.
- Flex your right foot to protect your knee joints.
- Inhale deeply to lengthen your spine.
- Exhale while gently pressing down on your right knee, feeling a stretch in your hip and outer thigh.
- Maintain a tall spine and relaxed shoulders as you deepen the stretch.
- Hold the pose for 15-30 seconds, breathing deeply and relaxing into the stretch.
- Inhale to relax the stretch, then exhale as you switch sides, putting your left ankle on top of your right thigh and repeating the stretch on the other side.

Reflection Box

Short description of how you felt during the pose and how you want to improve next time

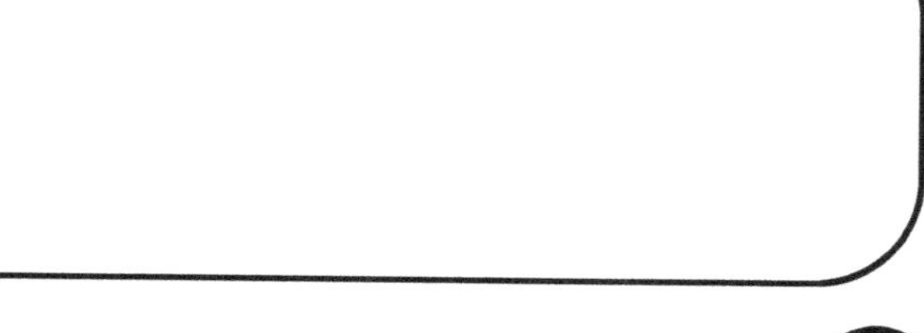

Seated Figure Four Stretch

- Sit comfortably in a chair, feet flat on the floor and spine upright.
- Lift your right foot from the ground and cross your right ankle over your left thigh.
- Flex your right foot to protect your knee joints.
- Inhale deeply to lengthen your spine.
- Exhale while gently pressing down on your right knee, feeling a stretch in your hip and outer thigh.
- Maintain a tall spine and relaxed shoulders as you deepen the stretch.
- Hold the pose for 15-30 seconds, breathing deeply and relaxing into the stretch.
- Inhale to relax the stretch, then exhale and switch sides, crossing your left ankle over your right thigh and repeating the stretch on the left side.

Reflection Box

Short description of how you felt during the pose and how you want to improve next time

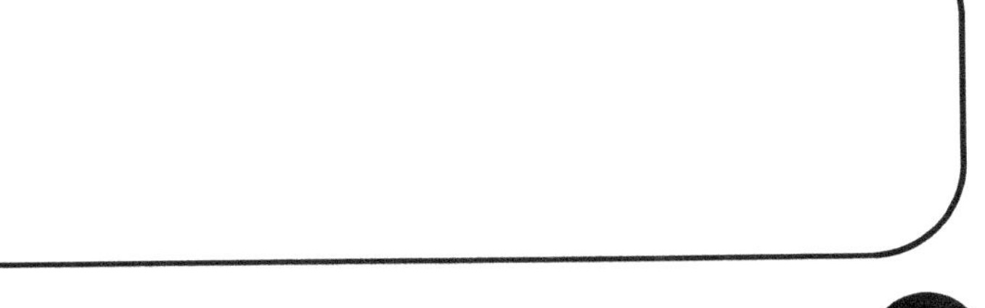

Seated Butterfly Stretch

- Sit comfortably in a chair, feet flat on the floor and spine upright.
- Bring the soles of your feet together, allowing your knees to extend to the sides.
- Hold your ankles or feet in your hands.
- Inhale deeply to lengthen your spine.
- Exhale as you gently press your knees down to the floor, feeling a stretch in your inner thighs and groin.
- Maintain a tall spine and relaxed shoulders as you deepen the stretch.
- Hold the pose for 15-30 seconds, breathing deeply and relaxing into the stretch.
- Inhale to release the stretch, then exhale to gently relieve pressure on your knees and return your feet to the floor.

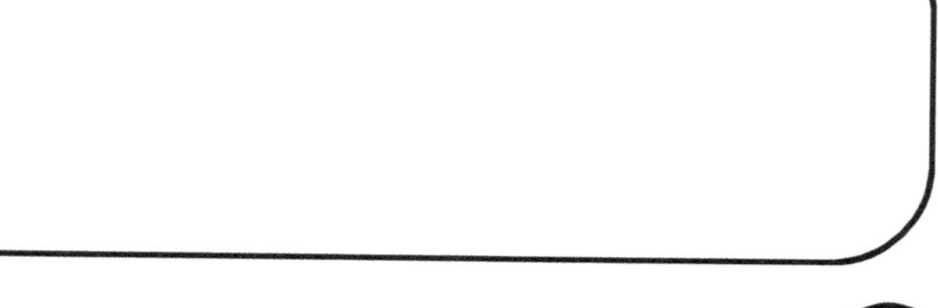

Reflection Box

Short description of how you felt during the pose and how you want to improve next time

Seated Hip Circles

- Sit comfortably in a chair, feet flat on the floor and spine upright.

- Put your hands on your knees for support.

- Prepare by inhaling deeply.

- Exhale as you move your hips to the right in a circular motion.

- Continue to circle your hips to the right for several rotations, moving smoothly and under control.

- Inhale as you finish the circles to the right.

- Exhale and reverse the direction of the circles, now circling your hips to the left.

- Continue to circle your hips to the left for several rotations, moving with your breath and paying attention to how your hips move.

Reflection Box

Short description of how you felt during the pose and how you want to improve next time

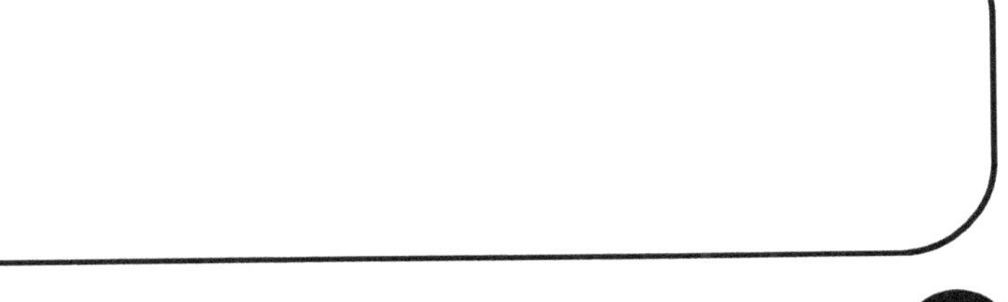

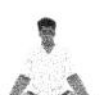

Chapter 11

Knees, Ankles, and Feet

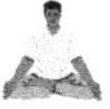

Seated Ankle Circles

- Sit comfortably in a chair, feet flat on the floor and spine upright.
- Lift your right foot off the ground and extend your right leg forwards.
- Rotate your right ankle in a clockwise direction.
- Make smooth and controlled circles starting at your ankle joint.
- After completing several rotations in one direction, switch to counterclockwise circles.
- Complete the ankle circles on your right foot, then repeat the process on your left.
- Continue alternating between both feet for several repetitions, moving with your breath and concentrating on loosening the ankle joints.

Reflection Box

Short description of how you felt during the pose and how you want to improve next time

Seated Knee-to-Chest Stretch

- Sit comfortably in a chair, feet flat on the floor and spine upright.
- Lift your right knee to your chest, gently hugging it with both hands.
- Keep your left foot flat on the ground and your spine upright.
- Hold the stretch for a few breaths to feel a gentle release in your hips and lower back.
- Inhale to lower your right leg to the floor.
- Repeat the stretch on the left side, bringing your left knee to your chest and holding for a few breaths.
- Continue alternating between both legs for several repetitions, moving with your breath and concentrating on the sensation of the stretch.

Reflection Box

Short description of how you felt during the pose and how you want to improve next time

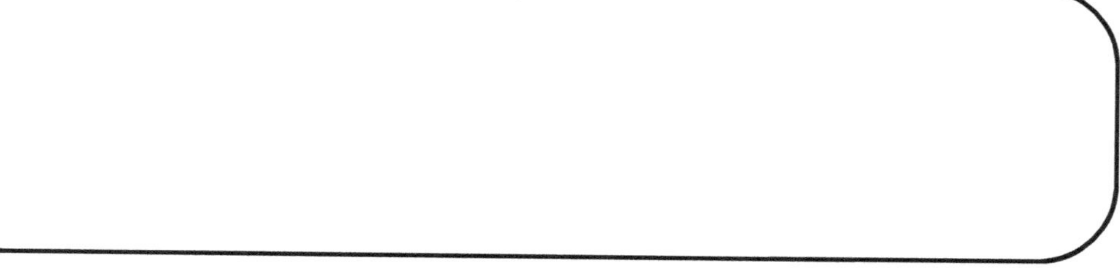

Seated Foot Flexor Stretch

- Sit comfortably in a chair, feet flat on the floor and spine upright.
- Extend your right leg forward, heel on the floor and toes pointing up at the ceiling.
- Gently pull back on your toes with your hands until you feel a stretch along the top of your foot and ankle.
- Hold the stretch for a few moments, taking deep breaths and relaxing into it.
- Release the stretch and switch to your left foot, extending it forward and flexing it.
- Pull back gently on your left toes, feeling a stretch along the top of your foot and ankle.
- Hold the stretch for a few moments, taking deep breaths and relaxing into it.
- Continue alternating between both feet for several repetitions, moving with your breath and concentrating on the sensation of the stretch.

Reflection Box

Short description of how you felt during the pose and how you want to improve next time

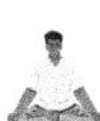

Seated Toe Point and Flex

- Sit comfortably in a chair, feet flat on the floor and spine upright.
- Extend your right leg forward, pointing your toes away from you, stretching the top of your foot and ankle.
- Hold the point for a few breaths and feel the gentle stretch.
- Flex your right foot, bringing your toes to your shin and stretching through the sole and ankle.
- Hold the flex for a few breaths until you feel a stretch on the bottom of your foot.
- Release the stretch and move to the left foot, pointing and flexing your toes in the same way.
- Continue to alternate pointing and flexing both feet for several repetitions, moving with your breath and concentrating on the sensation of the stretch.

Reflection Box

Short description of how you felt during the pose and how you want to improve next time

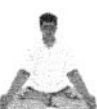

Seated Heel Raises

- Sit comfortably in a chair, feet flat on the floor and spine upright.
- Prepare by inhaling deeply.
- Exhale as you lift your heels off the ground and press into the balls of your feet.
- Hold the raised position for a moment while engaging your calf muscles.
- Inhale to bring your heels back to the ground.
- Repeat the heel raises several times, moving with your breath and concentrating on the contraction of your calf muscles.
- You can do the exercise with both feet at once or alternate between lifting each heel separately.

Reflection Box

Short description of how you felt during the pose and how you want to improve next time

Seated Ankle Alphabet

- Sit tall in a chair, feet flat on the floor, spine upright.
- Lift one foot off the floor while keeping the other grounded.
- Extend your lifted foot forward while keeping it flexed at the ankle.
- Imagine your big toe is a pencil, and "write" the letters of the alphabet in the air.
- Begin with the letter 'A' and progress through the alphabet, moving your ankle to form each letter.
- Keep your movements under control and precise as you trace each letter.
- After you've finished the alphabet with one foot, switch to the other and repeat the process.
- Take your time and move at a rate that allows you to precisely trace each letter.
- This exercise improves ankle mobility, strengthens the muscles surrounding the ankle joint, and enhances proprioception.

Reflection Box

Short description of how you felt during the pose and how you want to improve next time

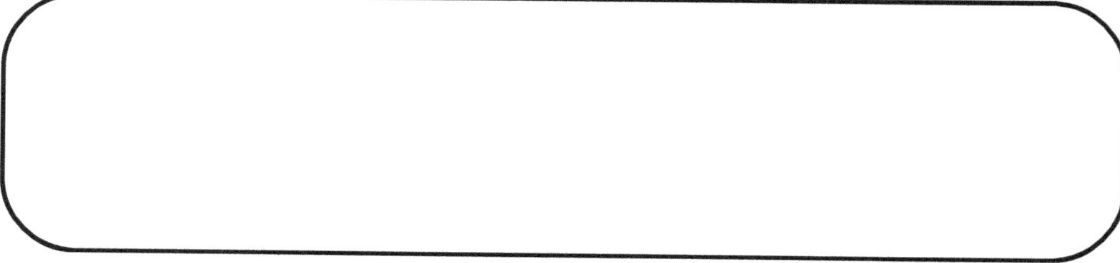

Chapter 12

Standing Poses with Chair

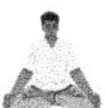

Chair Warrior I

- Sit at the front edge of a chair, feet flat on the floor, spine tall.
- Extend your right leg straight back behind you, toes on the floor, heel lifted.
- Bend your left knee, keeping it directly above your left ankle.
- Inhale as you raise your arms overhead and reach for the ceiling.
- Hold your torso upright and your shoulders relaxed.
- Sink into the stretch and feel a gentle opening in your hip flexors and calf muscles.
- Hold the pose for a few breaths, keeping your breathing steady.
- To release, exhale while lowering your arms and returning your right foot to the floor.
- Repeat the pose on the opposite side, extending your left leg back and bending your right knee.

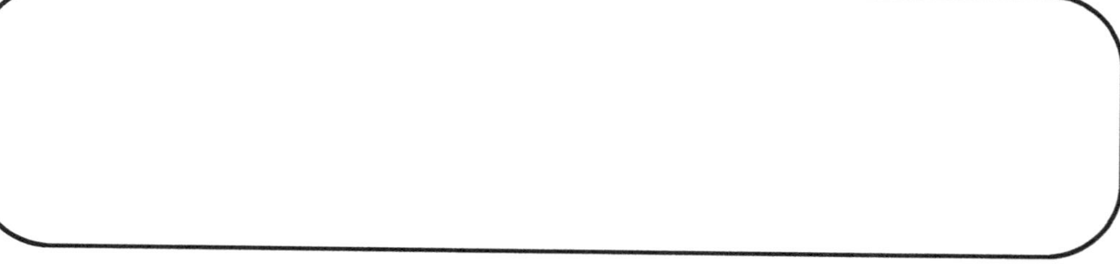

Reflection Box

Short description of how you felt during the pose and how you want to improve next time

Chair Warrior 2

- Sit at the front edge of a chair, feet flat on the floor, spine tall.
- Extend your right leg directly behind you and your left leg forward, keeping your feet hip-width apart.
- Rotate your right foot so it points to the side of the chair, while keeping your left foot pointed forward.
- Bend your left knee, keeping it directly above your left ankle.
- Inhale as you raise your arms parallel to the ground, fingertips away from one another.
- Keep your torso facing forward and your shoulders relaxed.
- Gaze over your left fingertips and feel a stretch in your inner thighs and sides of the torso.
- Hold the pose for a few breaths, keeping your breathing steady.
- To release, exhale while lowering your arms and returning your right foot to the floor.
- Repeat the pose on the opposite side, extending your left leg back and bending your right knee.

Reflection Box

Short description of how you felt during the pose and how you want to improve next time

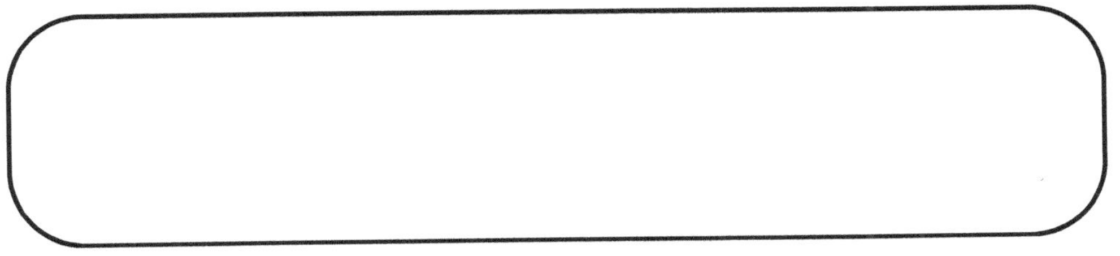

Chair Forward Fold

- Sit comfortably in a chair, feet flat on the floor and spine upright.
- Inhale deeply to lengthen your spine.
- Exhale as you bend forward from your hips and fold your torso over your thighs.
- Allow your arms to hang down to the floor, or reach for your feet or the chair legs.
- Keep your back straight and fold forward, leading with your chest.
- Relax your head and neck while feeling a stretch in your spine and the backs of your legs.
- Hold the forward fold for a few breaths before relaxing into the stretch.
- Inhale as you slowly lift your torso back to a seated position.

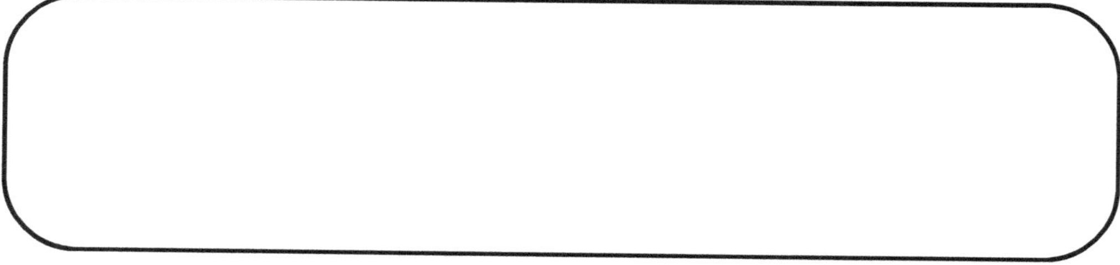

Reflection Box

Short description of how you felt during the pose and how you want to improve next time

Chair Tree Pose

- Sit comfortably in a chair, feet flat on the floor and spine upright.
- Move your weight to your left foot and lift your right foot off the ground.
- Place the sole of your right foot against the inside of your left calf or thigh, avoiding the knee joint.
- To create stability, press your foot into your leg, then your leg into your foot.
- Bring your hands to your heart center in a prayer position, or extend them overhead for an extra stretch.
- Find a focal point to help you balance, and then engage your core muscles.
- Hold the pose for a few breaths, feeling rooted and stable as a tree.
- To exhale, lower your right foot back to the floor.
- Repeat the pose on the opposite side, lifting your left foot and placing it against the inside of your right calf or thigh.

Reflection Box

Short description of how you felt during the pose and how you want to improve next time

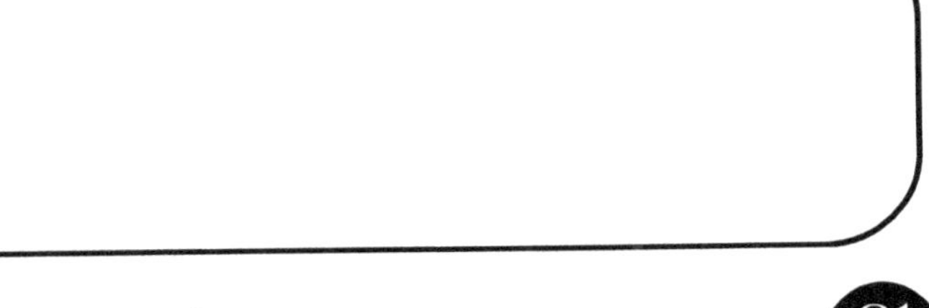

Chair Crescent Lunge

- Sit at the front edge of a chair, feet flat on the floor, spine tall.
- Extend your right leg straight back behind you, toes on the floor, heel lifted.
- Keep your left foot flat on the ground and your left knee bent directly over your left ankle.
- Inhale as you raise your arms overhead and reach for the ceiling.
- Sink into the stretch and feel a gentle opening in your hip flexors and calf muscles.
- Hold your torso upright and your shoulders relaxed.
- Hold the pose for a few breaths, keeping your breathing steady.
- To release, exhale while lowering your arms and returning your right foot to the floor.
- Repeat the pose on the opposite side, extending your left leg back and bending your right knee.

Reflection Box

Short description of how you felt during the pose and how you want to improve next time

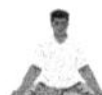

Conclusion

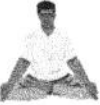

As we wrap up our journey through "Chair Yoga for Men Over 50," it's important to consider the practice's transformative power. Chair yoga provides a path to health, vitality, and well-being that is accessible to everyone, regardless of age or fitness level. We discovered how simple yet profound changes can occur within our bodies and minds by cultivating gentle movements, deep breathing, and mindful awareness in each session.

In a world that frequently expects more from us than we can give, chair yoga offers a respite—a place to pause, breathe, and reconnect with ourselves. It's more than just physical activity; it's about cultivating our inner landscape, finding peace in the midst of chaos, and embracing the entirety of our being.

Whether you want to relieve physical pain, improve your flexibility and strength, or simply find some peace in your hectic schedule, chair yoga can help. It's a practice that meets you where you're at, respecting your individual journey and encouraging you every step of the way.

So, as you continue your chair yoga journey, keep an open heart and a curious mind. Allow yourself to explore, grow, and discover the many benefits that this ancient tradition has to offer. And may the wisdom gained from your practice enrich every aspect of your life, bringing you joy, vitality, and radiant health for many years to come.

Testimonies

John, 57:

"Before I discovered chair yoga, I was struggling with chronic back pain and stiffness. But after incorporating the suggested exercises into my daily routine, I've experienced a significant reduction in discomfort and an increase in mobility. Chair yoga has truly been a game-changer for me, allowing me to reclaim my vitality and enjoy life to the fullest."

David, 62:

"I've always been skeptical of yoga, thinking it was only for flexible young people. However, after trying the exercises recommended in this book, I've been pleasantly surprised by how accessible and beneficial chair yoga can be. It's helped me manage stress, improve my balance, and even sleep better at night. I never imagined I'd become a yoga enthusiast at my age, but here I am, feeling healthier and happier than ever before."

Michael, 55:

"As someone who's never been particularly athletic, I was hesitant to try chair yoga. But thanks to the gentle guidance and encouragement provided in this book, I've discovered a newfound sense of strength and confidence in my body. The exercises have helped me feel more centered and at ease, both physically and mentally. I'm grateful for the opportunity to explore this practice and excited to see where it takes me in my journey toward optimal health and well-being."

WEEK 1   Chair Yoga Fitness Planner

DAY	EXERCISE	GOAL
Monday		
Tuesday		
Wednesday		
Thursday		
Friday		
Saturday		
Sunday		

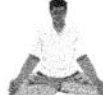

WEEK 2   Chair Yoga Fitness Planner

DAY	EXERCISE	GOAL
Monday		
Tuesday		
Wednesday		
Thursday		
Friday		
Saturday		
Sunday		

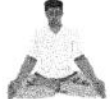

WEEK 3   Chair Yoga Fitness Planner

DAY	EXERCISE	GOAL
Monday		
Tuesday		
Wednesday		
Thursday		
Friday		
Saturday		
Sunday		

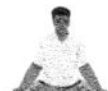

WEEK 4   Chair Yoga Fitness Planner

DAY	EXERCISE	GOAL
Monday		
Tuesday		
Wednesday		
Thursday		
Friday		
Saturday		
Sunday		

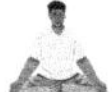

WEEK 5   Chair Yoga Fitness Planner

DAY	EXERCISE	GOAL
Monday		
Tuesday		
Wednesday		
Thursday		
Friday		
Saturday		
Sunday		

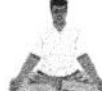